You Don't Loose Weight

How to Keep a *Successful* Weight Loss Diet

ELISABETH SETTER

Preface

Losing weight is one of the best value-for-effort actions a person can do, since it comes with very low or at no cost at all. Yet it is one of the most strenuous tasks to almost everyone.

Many types of weight-losing diets can be found, and the science behind it is becoming clearer every day. Still, it is beneficial for the general health and for the mental health of many, people find it hard to cope even with a non-drastic nutritional recommendation. Every dietary regime should be equilibrated, and a monotonous diet (a diet that contains only from one type of food) is usually not recommended by professionals.

In real life, it doesn't really matter what type of weight losing diet you may be on. There is a lot in common to the reasons you don't succeed in pursuing your goal. The basic rule in all diets is very simple - the balance between calories intake and output should always be negative. You can't drop those extra pounds if you add more than you subtract.

Other factors will influence the rate of losing weight, but the sheer facts you see every morning on the balance will result from calories gained versus calories spent. Whether you lost a half pound or 2 pounds (about 1 kg.) in a week depends not only by the calories, you entered your body but on other factors as your age and your personal metabolic rate (the rate that your body can use and store those calories) but the tendency toward losing or gaining weight is the mathematical result of calories in - calories out.

Being on weight-losing diet is like the rabbit and the turtle tale. The rabbit challenged the turtle to a race. While the rabbit ran fast and got exhausted soon, so he took a nap after a short distance while the turtle kept ongoing in his slow pace. When the rabbit woke up, he didn't see the turtle that already had reached the finish line, waiting for the arrogant rabbit there. It is to remember that racing on a weight-losing diet is much as the rabbit in this tale. You get exhausted, physically and mentally, quick and you may lose. Interest in keeping it. You'd rather go in a slow pace, all the way to the finish line.

Weight status is usually measured by calculating your BMI (Body-Mass-Index) that is a simple calculation that can be done by everyone. It is calculated by dividing your weight with the square root of your height. If you use Pounds and Inches the calculation is : 703 x weight (lbs) / [height (in]^2 . Using the metric system the formula is weight (kg) / [height (m)]^2 .

For example, if you are 64 inches tall and your weight is 140 pound, your BMI calculation will be: 730 x 140 / 64*64 (730 x 140 = 102,200) / (64 *64 = 4,096). Resulting in BMI of 24.9 . A 1.73 meter

tall and 72 kg in weight person has a BMI of 24.0
72 / (1.73*1.73) = 72/ 2.99 .

A BMI between 18.5 to 24.9 is considered normal
or healthy weight range; a BMI that is from 25 to
29.9 is considered overweight and a BMI 30 or
higher is defined as obesity.

Waist size is another important measurement that
is directly associated with an increased risk for
certain metabolic diseases. It is an independent
measurement and should not be confused with
BMI. It is possible to be at a normal BMI range
and still have an excess in undesired waist fat.

A waist larger than 94 cm (37 in) for Men and 80
(31.5 in) for Women is considered unhealthy and
can increase chances of diseases.

Those two measurements are easy to conduct
and together they can provide useful information
both on your weight losing success and on your
general risk.

Here are 10 most frequent reasons you don't lose weight and how to overcome them:

1. Medical issues

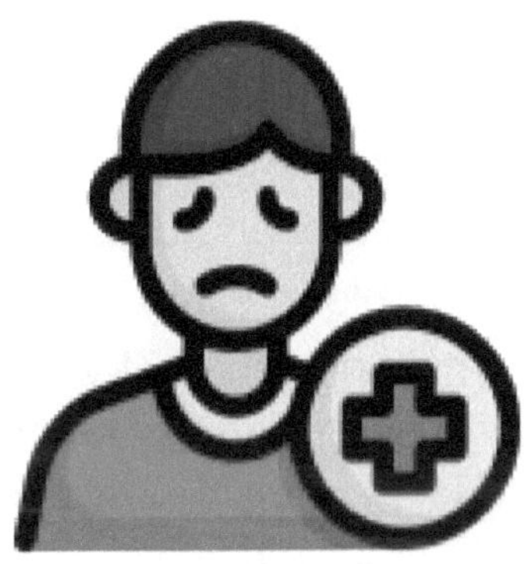

Not being able to lose weight, when you are in a low calories diet may be a warning sign for some health problem. One of the most common is a decreased function of the Thyroid gland. This gland, that is right in the middle of your neck, has the function to control your body metabolism, which is the rate your body absorbs food and turn them to energy. A decreased function of this gland may lead to slow metabolism, and therefore you may gain weight (and also be tired and loose hair). This disorder is mainly caused by an inflammation of the gland, but also people that went on surgery to remove the gland may be in the same situation if the medications they take are under the desired dose.

To verify if this is the cause you can't lose weight, consult with your doctor and do a blood exam. The most common blood exam to verify the possibility of a malfunctioning Thyroid is TSH (Thyroid-Stimulating Hormone). This hormone regulates the activity of the Thyroid and increased level of TSH means that the gland is performing too slow and vice versa.

Chronic stress can also interrupt your weight losing ambitions. If you are faced with a continuous stress, anxiety or grief your body may produce a certain hormone (cortisol to be exact) that causes your body to store more fat, and in particular belly fat. This kind of fat accumulation is often associated with a higher risk of diseases that are related to fat accumulation like Diabetes, high blood pressure and heart diseases. Waist circumference can be easily measured, but for itself it is not used to predict risk of diseases. Depression, that can be caused by a continuous stress or many other factors is often associated with being overweighted and have difficulties in losing weight. Depression can cause an excessive and unbalanced eating. Make sure that if you are in this situation get the best suitable treatment for this disease so that you'll be free to go with your weight losing ambitions.

Other potential medical conditions may be Diabetes mellitus and some other hormonal dysfunctions. Accumulation of water in the body, because of a disease or as a result of using certain medication, can also result in the inability to lose weight. In case you kept your low-calories diet vigorous, and you are sure that the total caloric intake (including those "little snacks") is less than what you use, visit your physician to check for the reason.

It's not only a medical condition that can make you gain weight, but also treatment for some illnesses do encourage weight gain. Corticosteroids, anti-Diabetes medications and some medications used in the treatment of psychiatric disorders can induce weight gain. If you feel that medications you take plays a role in your inability to loose weight, please consult your physician that may try to substitute them with others.

2. Over-compensation after workout

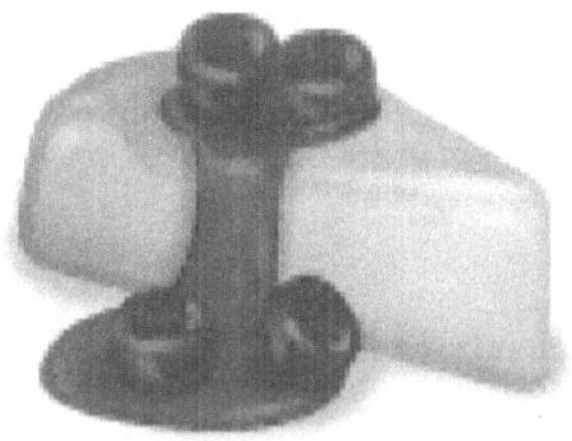

Physical activity has many benefits, including reducing your weight. It is a part of the balance of input and output of calories that can make you eliminate those unwanted pounds. We should remember that for most people, physical activity by itself is not the best strategy for losing weight. Walking for an entire hour at a moderate pace will burn 280 calories, same as one-hour biking. A medium-sized fresh Banana worth about 100 calories, one vegetable Egg Roll is about 150 calories and one slice of bread worth about 65.

"Burning calories" for the purpose of reducing weight is not necessarily the best strategy for losing weight, given the effort it takes. We should emphasize that being physically active is indeed important, but here we concentrate only on losing weight.

Some people misjudge the calorie balance (what gets in and what goes out) and "permit" themselves to overcompensate a workout with an amount of calories that is much more than those burned during the physical activity, and as a result - they not only avoiding a healthy weight reduction but may achieve the opposite result. One of the common "excuses" for this phenomenon is convincing yourself that the increased weight is due to "augmentation of the muscles" or "increasing muscle mass" and assuming that the weight gain is positive and demonstrate that your physical activity is beneficial (in the sense of weight control).

Just bear in mind that for a young male who does intensive training may gain 3-4 extra pounds in 3-4 months. Those figures depend on many other factors (hormonal status, having a good sleep, protein intake) so they can vary from one person to another, but can serve as a rule of thumb. If you are physically active and you gained more weight, please consider your total calories intake, and don't just assume its muscle mass.

Alcohol can also affect your weight loss efforts. Calories gained from alcohol are considered "empty" meaning they contain little nutrients. It is a good energetic source but it burns first, so your body uses it as a fuel rather that using its own accumulated fat, leaving it in your body. Depend on the amount. Alcohol can cause you to be unattended to what you eat and to the total calories that you take may be much higher than expected or planned. Another way alcohol can decrease your weight losing effort is by inhibiting testosterone levels in your body. This can result in slowing down the process. It can also increase your appetite too. It also decreases secretion of digestive juices from your liver and gallbladder that can result in poorer digestion. The last way alcohol can be an obstacle to dieting efforts is its relatively high content of calories, that you may not take inconsideration planning your daily diet.

3. You eat too little - Starvation mode

Putting your body in 'starvation mode' may lead to an undesirable response that is lowering your metabolism rate, a status that can prevent losing weight. When you don't give the body enough calories it needs, or if you are losing too much weight, the brain feels a sense of danger and reduces the number of calories it burns. It also may cause other symptoms like feel of hunger, weakness, fatigue and sometimes headache and it can make you feel weak. It is a natural defense mechanism of the body. As a result, the brain causes you hungrier, in order to "persuade" you to eat more and compensate for those calories and fat tissue lost, thus making you eat more calories that are needed. Another defense mechanism induced by the brain is slowing down metabolism, which makes the number of calories you burn much smaller.

The result is that you feel much weaker, you get hungrier and you eat more, and the final balance is in favor of calories coming into your body. A true 'starvation mode' is rare, and it implies a scant amount of calories intake, but a relatively low intake (about 1000-1200 calories a day) may also trigger those response mechanisms that will cause a slowdown of the metabolic processes.

Skipping a meal or two or fasting for a day every week won't trigger this body response, but an extreme diet would.

This phenomenon, which is very common in those who practice an extreme weight-losing diet, can be prevented by controlling the number of calories you take. Remember, the secret for a successful weight-reducing diet is to consume fewer calories than you burn, but don't go to the extreme in both directions.

4. Sleeping too little

Sleeping is one of the most important things for weight losing. An enjoyable sleep for an adult is bout 7 hours a night. When you sleep too little, you may skip exercise because of being too tired or grab an extra snack or a cappuccino (to wake you up). Your brain suffers as well, and the decisions he makes in this situation differ from when he is sharper. This can result in avoiding the healthy diet you were on and being tempted to foods you used to avoid. Studies showed that when your brain is not as sharp as usual, you tend to eat bigger portions, rich in carbohydrates.

You should consider a good sleep as an energy booster, keeping your metabolism active and your attitude sharp. On the metabolic level, sleep deprivation makes your brain feel danger and the release of cortisol, that is a stress signaling hormone. As a result of increase blood cortisol, the brain orders to reduce metabolism to conserve energy, and here we are at the same loop of stress-induced weight gain. Another hormonal pathway that may cause weight increase is the fact that sleeping too little causes the body's reaction to insulin to diminish. The inevitable result is that sugar and other foods that had to turn in energy, with the help of insulin, now turn into fat tissue.

First, you should understand that sleep deprivation can harm your efforts to lose weight (or to keep it once you've reached the desired weight). Try to make a bedtime ritual, shut down all potential distractions as your phone or computer, dim the lights and read something. After a brief period of rest, turn out the lights and help your body produce the natural sleep hormone that is melatonin. If you can't fall asleep, think of some natural herbal based syrup or pill like valerian or passiflora and don't forget not to drink any caffeine-containing drinks at least 4 hours before bedtime.

5. Sweetened beverages

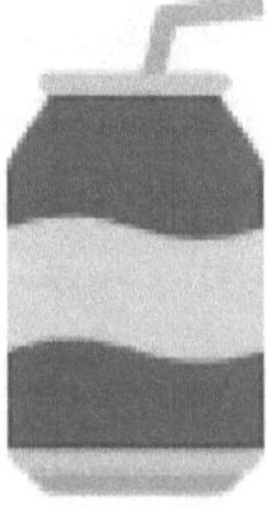

This is the leading source of added sugar in foods. Drinking sweetened beverages not only will ruin your efforts to lose weight but also may put you in a danger of serious diseases. Those beverages are associated with a greater chance of having diabetes, heart disease, kidney diseases or tooth decay and cavity. The source of those sugars (white or brown sugar, corn syrup, honey, malt syrup or others) does not substantially difference in their effect.

Data from the USA shows that over 60% of the young population doing a sweetened beverage on a daily basis and about 50% of adults. In the sense of calories, the average calories intake per day from those beverages amounts to 150. To have an idea, a teaspoon of white sugar contains about 15 calories and a tablespoon worth about 50 calories (that you can burn in 13 minutes of waking or 5 minutes of running).

Most beverages (in cans or personal bottles) will introduce to your body between 120 to 180 calories, only from that one drink. Remember that an average woman would need 1500 calories per day for a moderate weight losing diet and a similar man would need about 2000. Those sweetened beverages are added to the other beverage that may seem harmless. A cup of coffee with milk and sugar contains 65 calories, but one espresso with no milk or sugar has the value of 2.4 calories. A can of Sprite equals 140 calories, and a similar can of diet Sprite will have 0 calories.

It may sound not that high number of calories, but a single can-sized sweetened drink values 10% or more than your entire daily recommended calories intake (when you're on a weight losing diet).

6. Eating too much

This one may seem to be a simple and obvious one, but it is still the basis of weight losing diet. In order to lose weight, we need to reverse the caloric balance, i.e., to change the balance so that the calories we enter to our body will be less than those we take out. This is the only way to lose weight, and there are no shortcuts or alternatives. Yes, it is that simple equation, but yet so hard to achieve. So, how do we burn calories? The body has some constant activities that you cannot do without them, and they all (thankfully) consume energy and burn calories. Your heart is constantly beating, and your lungs gets and exhale air, so those are the two basic calories-expenditure processes. Other cells are on a continuous work like your liver, kidney and brain and they are also burning calories. Actually, the heart; brain; liver and kidney are in charge of about 65% of burning calories, even if you do nothing. We call it the basic metabolic rate and you can calculate it by yourself by a non-very complicated equation.

It is calculated that the average basal metabolic rate (BMR) is about 1,800 for an average male and 1,400 for a female. By defining "average male" or female we take the example of a 25-year-old male, 5.7 feet tall, weighting 165 pounds (1.75 meters, 75 kg). He has a basal metabolic rate of approximately 1,775 calories per day. The same male when he is 40 years of age will have a BMR of 1,670, and at the age of 60 the basal metabolic rate will decrease to 1,530. The equivalent women at a height of 5.6 feet weighting 143 pounds (1.7 m, 65 kg) will have a BMR of 1,470 at 25 years of age, 1,400 and 1,300 at ages of 40 and 60, respectively.

A simple way to calculate the BMR in accordance to your activity is to add 20% of calories burned when you have little or no exercise, 50% if you are physically active 3-5 days a week and 70% more for a very active person. If a 40-year-old woman that has a basal metabolic rate will be moderately active, she will burn 2,100 calories every day instead of 1,400 calories every day if she wasn't active.

Given those simple rules now, the question is how we can eat less. The thing here is all about being aware and planning in advance. When you plan your meal ahead, and you don't eat emotionally. You have a better control of what and how much you put into your body. Use smaller plates and bowls. Yes, it's all psychology here.

By decreasing the size of the plate its content seems bigger (because it makes it look full), that will satisfy your (hungry) brain that there is enough there and will help you feel full. Another way to eat less is by eating slowly and being concentrated on the process of eating. Take away any distraction like playing or reading news or answering e-mails while you eat or watching TV. Respect the "ceremony" of eating so you will not eat much more than you need. Eating in a slow pace will make you feel full earlier and you can spare some extra unneeded calories. Try eating more vegetables as they are usually poor in calories and will still make you feel full.

7. Boring physical activity

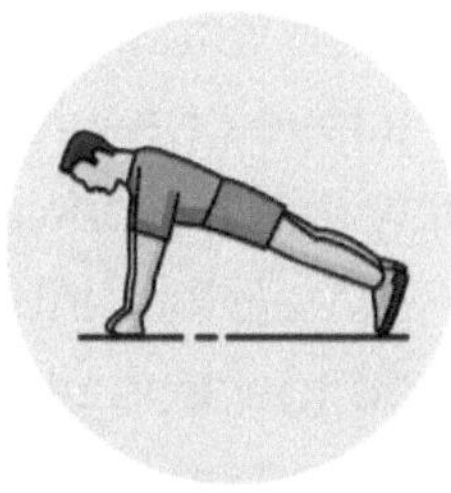

So, you are doing your best to be physically active and you do it at least three times a week, but you start shortening the sessions and you're happy to have some excuse to skip training. If this is your situation - you should be more creative in what you do.

Not all people love being physically active and when you try something new for you should be exited, or .. at least not bored. The best physical activity for you is the one you'll have fun to do and maintain. Don't rush and don't expect to have that beautiful body you wish instantly. Remember the tale of the rabbit and the turtle, the turtle always wins. The basics of a durable physical activity is planning, so you won't fall in that old excuse of "I don't have enough time". You always have time to what is important to you, so prioritize. Try to exercise with a friend or a family member or someone you like to be with. You will earn both a pleasing time with a love one while benefiting from the activity. You may join a workout group, so you'll get to know some other interesting people. Change your attitude towards physical activity, it really doesn't have to be dull or painful. Know your limits and understand that improvements come with time.

The more you exercise, the easy it will be and then you can set yourself a new goal. Consider using equipment at home, like a treadmill, so you can continue your activity in wintertime. Don't fall into common excuses not to exercise. See your goal and pursue it. A wristwatch or band can monitor your achievements and they are cheap these days. Set some goals (7,500 steps a day, for instance) and in a second time adjust them. This will keep you committed to yourself and to your goals.

8. Pendulum diet

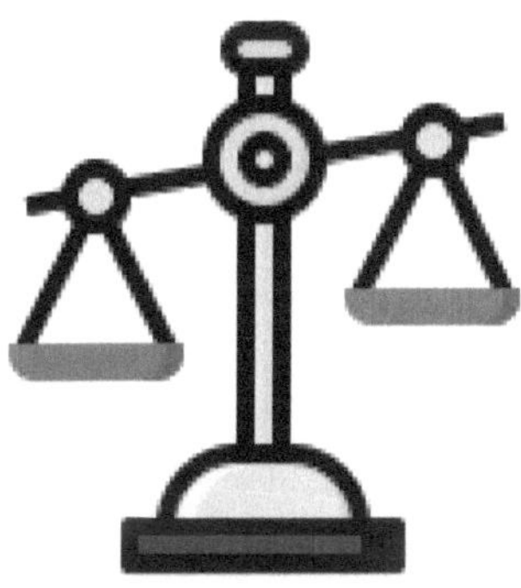

Going to extremes is not beneficial in many aspects of life, and a diet of one week "eat as you can" and the next one of starvation, will do more harm than good to your body and your efforts of losing weight. You should remember that when you go to the extremes on one side you may find yourself at the opposite extreme later.

Many people on a rigorous diet tend to "give up" after a brief period of time and compensate themselves by overeating. The pendulum effect combines both the starvation mode and overcompensation. The brain gets confused – on one side it slows the metabolism because of the starvation effect and next it has to deal with the excess of calories, which turns out a defensive mechanism. This mechanism causes that the metabolism rate is being slowed also in the overeating period, which aggravates the caloric imbalance.

The thing with weight losing diet is to proceed in a slow pace and not to make rapid changes. This is the 'secret' for a successful weight losing.

People nowadays search for instant rewards, but your body and your brain have evolved over thousand years to make slow changes. You shouldn't challenge them to change their habits, you won't succeed!

9. You don't feel that you really need to lose weight

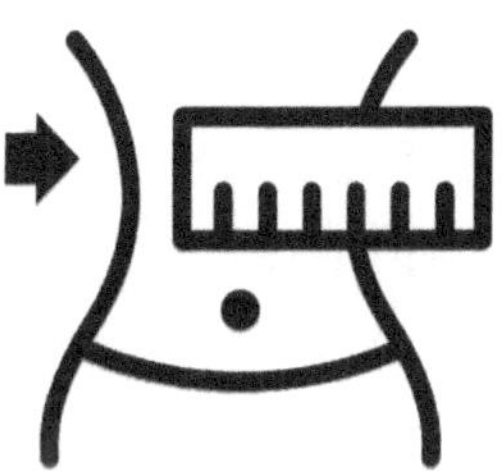

That is fine, too. But are you honest with yourself? You may think you need not lose weight because you are already at the ideal weight, everyone adores your body and you feel up in the sky. It all depends on your body image. You may be happy with your weight, even if it's out of the "standards".

Remember that the perception of weight, and what is right and what is wrong, is subjective and changes between societies. You cannot only rely on what is "recommended" as the ideal weight for you. In several societies being, what they usually call "overweighted" is the norm. Other societies encourage women to be overweighted and consider it as being more healthy than lean women.

You don't have to lose weight unless it comes from you, and you are the one that decided to begin a weight losing diet. That said, it is always good to remember that some physical activity is always beneficial. Engage in a moderate activity that will help your body be more flexible and strengthen your muscles. Those exercises (including Yoga or Pilates) will keep your body in a good shape and may prevent all kinds of aches, like backache or muscle pain, will make you stand and walk in a straighter position and will help you feel more confident.

10. You don't drink enough water

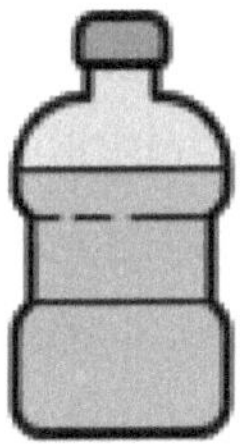

Simple as it sounds, the scent of life, or pure water is one secret for a successful weight losing diet.

When your stomach is full, it expands and receptors that are in the stomach's wall sense it. They signal the brain saying that all is OK, and you feel full. So why not 'trick' those sensors and fill the stomach with zero-calories? Many medical studies have proven the fact that drinking water prior to a meal reduces the amount of calories in that meal (just because you eat less) and a reduction in body weight.

It also seems that drinking water can increase calories burning, and in particular drinking chilly water. Yes, it's not that much of calories, but in order to heat the water inside your body some extra calories will go away.

Another benefit gained from drinking pure water is the fact that you won't drink sweetened drinks, and thus you have spared (probably many) calories. The same rule is true for drinking non-sweetened tea or herbal infusions, if you like them more.

Don't exaggerate in drinking water. Remember that weight losing is all about a delicate balance between your personal body's needs and what you give it. As a rule of thumb, 8 glasses of water should be sufficient for the average adult. If you live in a very hot climate, or do a physical effort for living, you'd need some more. Drinking too much water can harm as it dilutes the salts in your blood and more precisely the levels of sodium. A low sodium level can result in headache, weakness, muscle cramps or even confusion.

www.ingramcontent.com/pod-product-compliance
Lightning Source LLC
Chambersburg PA
CBHW031922270726
48655CB00007BA/3138